Wall Pilates Workouts for Women

"Strengthen Your Core, Sculpt Your Body, and Transform Your Posture with Wall Pilates"

Emma Stone

Table of Contents

Introduction 4

Chapter 1 History of Pilates..7

Chapter 2: Getting Started 10

    Principles of Pilates: 10

    Why Choose Pilates? 12

    Choosing a Pilates Instructor 14

Chapter 3: Equipment Needed 18

    Essential Equipment for Wall Pilates 18

    Alternatives and DIY Options 19

    Tips for Using Alternatives and DIY Equipment 21

    Advantages of Pilates in Pregnancy 22

Chapter 4: Basic Wall Pilates Exercises 27

    Warm-Up Exercises 27

    The Hundred 27

    Chest Lift 28

    Roll-Up 29

    Rolling Like a Ball 29

    One-Leg Circle 30

    Open Leg Balance 31

    Plank Pose 31

    The Side Kick Series 32

    Kick Front 32

Single Leg Stretch 33

Spine Stretch 34

Double Leg Stretch 34

The Saw 35

The Swan 35

Pilates Push-up 36

Chapter 5: Intermediate Wall Pilates Exercises 37

Wall Plank 37

Wall Bridge 38

Wall Push-Ups 40

Chapter 6: Advanced Wall Pilates Exercises 42

Wall Pike 42

Wall Scissors 43

Chapter 7: Beyond Exercise E-book 47

Diet Plan 47

Workout Plan 52

Breathing Techniques 59

Conclusion 62

Introduction

Put yourself in this situation: it has been a long day, you have been slumped over a computer for hours, your neck is tight, and the idea of going to the gym seems like it would be tiresome. The gym is like a terrifying jungle, filled with intricate machinery and people who are so fit that they are intimidating. There are countless ladies who go through the same struggle on a daily basis, and you are not the only one who feels this way. What if there was a method to completely modify your typical training regimen, find relief from discomfort, and attain the toned and flexible physique you have always dreamed of, all without leaving the convenience of your own home? Introducing Wall Pilates, a cutting-edge method of physical exercise that promises to completely transform the way you enjoy your workout classes.

We are all aware of the difficulties that come with living in the current world. A lack of time for self-care is frequently a consequence of juggling the demands of job, family, and personal life. Traditional workouts can feel like a chore because they need not just time but also mental energy to traverse busy gyms or follow detailed routines. This can make traditional exercising feel like a chore. The frustration that comes from not getting the results that they want despite their best efforts is something that many women go through. There is a possibility that you are fighting with recurrent aches and pains, or that you are having difficulty persevering through a fitness regimen that simply does not appear to be able to accommodate your hectic schedule.

It is the purpose of this book to alter that. A comprehensive solution that is geared to match your specific requirements, "Wall Pilates Workouts for Women" is more than simply a fitness guide; it is an all-encompassing solution. Wall Pilates is a form of exercise that takes the power of Pilates, which is a discipline that is well-known for its emphasis on core strength, flexibility, and conscious movement, and mixes it with the support and stability of a wall. The combination of these two factors results in an exercise that is not only effective but also available to people of varying fitness levels.

Imagine a workout that does not require expensive equipment, that would allow you to perform it in the comfort of your own living room, and that would target all of the appropriate muscles while also enhancing your posture and providing pain relief. These benefits, along with many others, are offered by wall Pilates. Through the incorporation of the wall into your routine, you will acquire a trustworthy companion in your road toward fitness. This companion will assist you in maintaining good form, improving your balance, and boosting your self-confidence.

Within the pages of "Wall Pilates Workouts for Women," you will find a methodical strategy to adopting Wall Pilates into your everyday practice. The book is broken up into pieces that are simple to understand and follow, and each of these sections is intended to make the process of mastering this transforming practice easier for you.

All of the exercises in "Wall Pilates Workouts for Women" were designed with you in mind. For years, the author, who is a seasoned Pilates instructor and fitness lover, has been assisting women like you in transforming their bodies and lives through the power of Pilates. As a result of the author's profound comprehension of the typical obstacles that women have while attempting to keep up with a regular fitness regimen, the author has developed a program that is not only efficient but also entertaining and environmentally friendly.

The author's expertise is supported by years of training, certifications, and practical experience obtained via hands-on work. Due to the fact that she has worked with women of varying ages and fitness levels, the author is aware of what is successful and what is not. This book condenses that information into a handbook that is not only easy to understand but also practical and applicable to everybody. In order to ensure that any woman, regardless of where she is in her fitness journey, is able to reap the benefits of Wall Pilates, the routines have been created to be inclusive.

It is important to keep in mind that the key to success resides in maintaining consistency and being conscious as you embark on your path. This book is not about quick solutions or making promises that are impossible to keep; rather, it is about developing a practice that is environmentally friendly and improves your quality of life in general. It is not necessary for you to have to spend a lot of time at the gym or purchase expensive equipment. You only need a wall, a little bit of space, and a commitment to yourself in order to pull this off.

You should begin with the fundamentals, take your time to fully comprehend each workout, and then gradually build up your overall regimen. Pay attention to what your body is telling you, have patience with yourself, and delight in each and every minor triumph along the path. You will be able to observe and experience the transformation going on in both your body and mind if you are dedicated and have the appropriate instruction.

By selecting "Wall Pilates Workouts for Women," you are making a constructive move toward improved health and well-being for yourself and your family. This book will be your travel companion on the path to becoming a more powerful, versatile, and self-assured version of yourself. It will be easier for you to overcome challenges, maintain your motivation, and accomplish your fitness objectives if you follow the author's guidance, which is straightforward, encouraging, and expert.

Imagine that you already have more energy, that you have better posture, and that you are able to move through your day with ease and grace. Imagine having a body that not only looks fantastic but also feels powerful and capable of doing whatever you want it to. This book is designed to assist you in turning the promise of Wall Pilates into a reality, and it is here to accomplish that promise.

Are you prepared to make significant changes to both your workout program and your life? It's time to get started.

Chapter 1 History of Pilates

Joseph Pilates, a physical therapist from Germany, is credited for developing the great Pilates workout regimen. The gymnast who was his father was a well-known figure in Greek gymnastics, and his mother was a naturopath. Over the course of his life, he learned both Western and Eastern mind-body exercises in attempt to improve his physical health and overcome ailments such as asthma. The concept of a man who embodies a harmonious body, mind, and spirit was a significant impact on him. This concept originated in Greek philosophy. In order to extend his awareness, he participated in a variety of physical activities, including yoga, gymnastics, boxing, skiing, diving, and others. In addition to this, he investigated the movements of animals in order to comprehend their proper form.

It was in the early years of the 20th century when Joseph first started developing his own personal fitness routine. He believed that mental and physical health were inextricably linked, and as a result, his primary purpose was to improve both the physical and mental aspects of one's health. Through the utilization of a variety of instruments that he referred to as "Apparatus," he developed methods that assisted individuals in accelerating the process of aligning, stretching, and strengthening various parts of their bodies. The individual made an attempt to develop a variety of routines that will enable the body to perform at its highest potential.

In 1912, Joseph made the journey to England in order to find employment as a self-defense instructor. Because he was considered an enemy alien during World War I, he was held in detention alongside other German nationals. During his time in prison, he utilized his training routine to instruct the other people who were being held as interns. However, not a single one of Joseph's trainees passed away during the influenza epidemic that occurred in 1918 and took thousands of lives. After being released from prison, he went back to Germany, where the dance community, in particular, enthusiastically accepted his exercises. Since Rudolf von Laban is responsible for the creation of a dance notation that is still utilized today, we are grateful to him. Joseph's methods were later used into a variety of dance curriculum, including one that was developed by Hanya Holm. After receiving a request from representatives of the

German government to use his fitness routine to train the military, Joseph took the choice to leave Germany permanently.

Joseph made his way to the United States of America in 1926, the same year that he met Clara, the woman who would become his partner. Following that, the couple tied the wedding and opened a fitness center in New York City that they named "Studio for Body Contrology" together. The New York City Ballet was represented by a large number of dancers and ballerinas who were among their clients. The number of dancers who visited his studio increased after they learned that Pilates may assist in the development of a body that is robust, lean, and healthy. Some of Joseph's students were well-known boxers, opera singers, merchants, veterans of war, and a great number of other notable individuals. The Pilates method gained popularity not only in New York City but also in other places. Additionally, this particular exercise routine was utilized by thousands of elementary school students all across the world.

At the same time, Joseph's students began passing on his exercise routine, which led to an increase in its popularity across the country. The two individuals who were responsible for establishing their own Pilates studios and teaching the method were Bob Seed and Carola Trier. Carola was a professional contortionist, and Bob had a history of playing hockey in several incarnations. Additionally, Joseph and Clara were acquainted with numerous choreographers, including the well-known George Balanchine, who was one among their many contacts.

When Joseph Pilates went away in 1967, there was no succession plan in place for the Pilates business whatsoever. Unfortunately, he did not appoint somebody to carry on his lessons, and he lacked the will to do so. Despite this, he continued to facilitate the operation of his workshop in New York with the assistance of his partner Clara and a handful of his students. Around the year 1970, Romana Kryzanowska, who had previously been a student of Joe and Clara, assumed the role of director. His students began opening their own studios and teaching Pilates, and the number of his students who did so continued to rise.

The 1980s marked the beginning of the media's coverage of Pilates. Its popularity spread across the world as a result of the participation of a large number of famous people in the practice. Pilates is a form of exercise that has gained popularity throughout the course of time. Pilates is currently being done by millions of people all around the world, and the number of people working out with Pilates is continuously growing.

The fact that there are currently a great number of excellent training programs accessible does not change the fact that some of these programs produce instructors who are not qualified because of their streamlined and standardised curriculums. There has also been an increase in the expense of training; currently, mat exercises cost between $10 and $20 per hour, while employing Pilates equipment costs between $50 and $100 per hour. The Pilates Method Alliance was founded in 2001 with the purpose of promoting and upholding the commitment to train Pilates instructors. This is due to the belief that having teachers who are both knowledgeable and well-trained is necessary in order to assist students in reaching their full potential. The Pilates Examination Exam was first developed by the organization in 2005 with the purpose of evaluating a teacher's level of expertise in the field of Pilates. At the moment, there are a great number of competent teachers spread all over the world, and a rising number of individuals are making an effort to accept the practice's level of competency and safety.

Chapter 2: Getting Started

Pilates is a complete synchronization and dexterity of soul, mind, and body, or contrology, as its creator advocated. Pilates practitioners learn to firmly and efficiently regulate every movement and function of their bodies during their training. This control and management is then applied to gain the synchronization of soul and subconscious activity. A healthy and tranquil body is the ultimate outcome when all the many domains of the body and soul are operating under the same synchronization and harmony.

But in order for repeated Pilates practice to help you reach your goals, all of this harmonization and management calls for constancy and a strong feeling of will.

Pilates is the most well-known and successful method for regaining physical vitality, improving mood, promoting body health, and correcting unbalanced body postures. These traits are essentially innate to the human body during the earliest stages of infancy, when the body and soul have the same, efficient, and coherent directives. But as the child progressively approaches maturity and begins to encounter the harsh and brutal truths of life, this innocence and synchronicity are quickly lost. The human body's physical clothing is the first thing to suffer throughout this difficult struggle with life's reality. Wearied eyes, callused crow's feet, tense shoulders, and hazy postures are some physical signs of the aftereffects. Many believe it to be the effects of getting older, but this is untrue as becoming older does not necessarily imply poor health. All we have to do is get our bodies back to its former vigor and rigor while nurturing our spirits and treating ourselves like priceless gems, which is ultimately what makes us successful. One method that will help you restore your body's power and muscles is Pilates.

Principles of Pilates:

In spite of the fact that we have been discussing how the area of Pilates technique for body stability has become so broad that numerous additions, adjustments, and variations have made it a more helpful approach, there are some Pilates principles that involve the central ideas of these techniques.

- **Concentration**

Focusing is the most important thing. When we are so overburdened with work-related expectations and deadlines, many of you may be wondering how it is possible to maintain attention in this situation. Consequently, the approaches that Pilate employs are beneficial to you in terms of developing and mastering the ability to concentrate. The ability to concentrate is absolutely necessary in order to achieve the objective of Pilate's fitness program, which is to alleviate the individual of tension and issues. These exercises have the potential to improve attention, which in turn can make it easier for the practitioner to forget about their troubles and concentrate on their workout. Once the desired level of focus has been attained, the particular results of utilizing this method will become readily obvious.

- **Control**

Control is defined as the capacity to exert or exert control over one's own movements, muscular strengths, and patterns of movement within the body. At the same time as these concepts constitute the sequential steps of Pilate's approach, they are also intricately connected to one another. An excessive amount of focus and concentration will, in the long run, result in the management and control of the body. There are probably a lot of you who have thought about how important control is. Considering that the main concept behind Pilates is to provide individuals the opportunity to experience the controllability of their own body movements and postures, Pilates will be of great assistance to you in learning this.

- **Centering**

Pilates workout routines concentrate an emphasis on beginning in a centered stance or starting from a certain spot. As the principal aim for bodily movements and the management point, the middle abdomen has been positioned as the primary target by the majority of perspectives on the center. As a consequence of this, the entire system of limbs and abdominal muscles is maintained in a highly focused manner in order to serve as the center of rigor and strength respectively.

- **Precision**

Among all the components, precision is the most crucial and significant one. Due to the fact that the human body is also prone to making mistakes, the precise planning of the entire study plan, which included the activities and posters, was carried out with full accuracy. When it comes to poor body alignment and movement, the human body can be fragile, despite the fact that it is designed to be powerful and robust. As a result, Pilates instructors often take this aspect into consideration and modify each exercise to cater to the specific preferences and capabilities of each individual student. A slight disregard for the specific needs of each individual human body can substantially damage the precision of exercise, making it hard to account for the positive impacts that exercise has. With regard to the physical output, precision might not appear to be all that significant to the normal person; nonetheless, it is the foundation of Pilates.

- **Power house**

A further distinctive feature of this physical exercise and output scheme is that it places an emphasis on the power house in connection to the human body as a set of organs that work together in harmony. According to the Pilates philosophy, the power house of the human body is positioned at the center of the structure of the human body. As a consequence, the consolidation of this formidable force is the ultimate consequence of all of the essential concepts that were mentioned before.

Why Choose Pilates?

To develop and tone your muscles, there are a multitude of various workouts that you may choose from. These workouts claim to help you achieve your goals. Why should you choose Pilates instead of one of these other options when you have had the opportunity to try out or learn about a couple of them?

The following are some of the elements that will contribute to the significance of Pilates for you.

Build Up the Whole Body

When you go to the gym, you could find that you engage in more physical activity in one particular region of your body than in the others. It is simple to concentrate on developing your biceps and triceps while ignoring your thighs and calves. This is because strengthening your arms is a simple exercise. You become disproportionate as a result of this, and much worse, you get unsatisfied with your physical look.

Pilates is a form of exercise that targets every part of your body from head to toe since it has a strong emphasis on strengthening your core.

As a result of the fact that everything begins at the core, Pilates teaches your body to work as a complete rather than just a particular location. An increase in general strength as well as a better degree of body flexibility is encouraged. Increasing the strength of your joints is the objective of Pilates.

A further discovery you will make is that Pilates is beneficial to the growth of your mind. In this way, Pilates might have an effect on your mental state. One of the things that Pilates needs of you is to pause and focus your attention on the individual motions and exercises that you are performing. In order to allow your body and mind to relax, you need to take long, deep breaths and hold them for a considerable amount of time. In a way that other forms of exercise would not, this improves one's fitness level.

Many Learning Methods

Taking private sessions from a Pilates instructor would be the ideal method to begin learning Pilates. By getting to know yourself and your body, you can design workouts that will strengthen you and improve your chances of success. If you want to profit from Pilates but lack the funds to see an instructor, what should you do?

There are exercises like this one that are simple to learn. You can try to educate yourself the methods whenever it's convenient for you. What you require are the appropriate starting supplies and clothing.

To start, all you'll need is a Pilates mat. You may then simply follow online training videos from that point on. As with this ebook, you might also purchase some books and study the moves. Pilates is not tough, but it can be challenging to do it incorrectly.

For the Pilates Body

Individuals who practiced Pilates had bodies that were more toned, better aligned, and even smaller. By focusing on the core of the body, one can attain the best results in terms of improving their breathing and circulation. People who do Pilates breathing exercises are more likely to slow down their activities, which is beneficial to the circulatory system of the cardiovascular system. When it comes to the Pilates body, aesthetics and look are not the only elements to consider. Furthermore, there is the benefit of the way that it operates on the inside.

Due to the fact that the blood gets detoxified from all of the oxygen that it is exposed to, Pilates is an extremely effective method for promoting blood circulation. Because of this, the system is revitalized, and the natural rhythm within the body is enhanced.

An additional advantage is that the workouts give you a more flexible spine, which is a result of the strengthening of your spine. Specifically, this is due to the fact that the exercises improve the alignment of all of the bones in the body, as the core muscles are responsible for supporting the spine.

People who have been doing Pilates for a significant amount of time and who have experienced back pain will attest to the benefits that they have obtained.

Choosing a Pilates Instructor

Starting out with a Pilates instructor who can walk you through all of the essential exercises and show you the ropes is the best way to get started with Pilates. Due to the fact that Pilates is founded on scientific principles, it is absolutely necessary for your instructor to have a substantial amount of understanding regarding the entire system of exercises. Your instructor should not only be able to provide you with quality teaching, but they should also be able to explain the duties that were assigned to you in a clear and concise manner. The level of achievement that you desire to accomplish as a Pilates student will be significantly impacted by the experience that you have achieved in the past.

This chapter contains a few suggestions that provide guidance on how to locate the most suitable instructor.

Find out about Pilates

There is no such thing as a Pilates training routine in which you go to the studio, finish a short lesson, and then go. The nature of the labor is hard, and it necessitates a detailed approach to do the work. For you to be able to determine whether or not the exercises are beneficial to you, it is required for you to begin with a predetermined number of sessions. After that, you will be able to make another determination.

It is therefore necessary for you to hire a Pilates instructor who has a significant amount of experience and training in the field. At the very least, you should be sure that your instructor has undergone 450 hours of intensive Pilates instructor training.

Clarity of Instruction

It is necessary for you to have an understanding of what your instructor is saying in order to correctly follow their directions. Before making any decisions, you should attend one of their workshops and watch what they demonstrate. Proceed to someone whose directions and communication are easy to understand if you realize that you are finding yourself a little confused, even if it is simply by viewing.

Professionalism and Confidence

Given that you and your instructor will be working together, it is the responsibility of both of you to ensure that they behave themselves in a manner that is highly professional. There will be moments when your instructor will need to touch you; in these circumstances, you should never have the impression that the instructor is acting in an inappropriate manner. Talking to other students and observing how comfortable they are is the most effective way to evaluate the level of professionalism that is present in the classroom.

Enjoyable and Motivational

Because Pilates is not a form of exercise that is intended to produce discomfort, it is presumed that you had a good time during your Pilates class. It is the responsibility of your instructor to inspire you to take pleasure in the activities you are participating in. In addition to this, you need to be motivated, which may be accomplished by having your instructor check in with you to ensure that the class is proceeding as planned and that you are not experiencing any discomfort or suffering.

Meeting your Needs

Before you begin a Pilates session, it is essential that your Pilates instructor takes the time to assess your requirements and devise a workout routine that is tailored to your specific demands. For this reason, you should be sure that your Pilates instructor is teaching the conventional Pilates method in the way that it was intended to be taught. There are various novel approaches that have not yet been thoroughly tried and verified. In addition, you need a teacher who demonstrates a real concern for assisting you in accomplishing your goals, as evidenced by the manner in which they conduct themselves.

The Mind Should Be in Focus

Not only does Pilates provide a workout for the body, but it also helps to create some mental equilibrium, which is an additional benefit of practicing Pilates. It is expected that the instructor will be able to achieve this level of equilibrium by including some form of movement meditation into the exercises that you will be practicing. In the event that you discover that your instructor is just interested in putting you through a variety of new exercises and experimenting with a variety of different props, you should consider switching to someone else who is better able to match your requirements.

Variety is Key

Every time you go to a Pilates class, in addition to the exercises that are considered to be staples, you should also be introduced to new exercises. It would be more beneficial for you to be engaged in a learning process rather than being immersed in an experience that is oriented on routine and repetition. There is no need for you to be concerned about reaching a plateau in your workout program because your instructor should have no trouble incorporating new workouts into your routine. If there are not too many new exercises being taught, then at the very least, there should be some modifications made to the exercises that are considered to be more conventional.

Certification

In addition to having the requisite qualifications to instruct Pilates, your instructor is required to hold certification from a body that is both recognized and certified. Even if a person has personal experience doing Pilates on their own, this does not mean that they are qualified to instruct others in the approach. It is essential to have someone who is not only knowledgeable about Pilates but also has possibly had extra training in other forms of movement, such as yoga instruction. In this manner, your body will experience the most possible benefits.

Chapter 3: Equipment Needed

For wall Pilates, which is an approachable and effective form of Pilates, the equipment required to get started is straightforward. In this chapter, you will be guided through the necessary equipment, several options will be discussed for various price ranges, and do-it-yourself solutions will be provided for those individuals who would prefer to construct their own equipment or use what they were already in possession of.

Essential Equipment for Wall Pilates

1. **Wall Space**

Naturally, a wall is the most important "piece" of equipment in Wall Pilates. Make sure you have a stretch of wall space that is free of obstacles, such as furniture, windows, or photos. You should be able to sustain your body weight on the wall while performing different workouts.

2. **Exercise Mat**

A nonslip and cozy surface for floor activities is offered by an exercise mat. Pick a mat that provides enough padding to keep your spine and joints safe. High-density foam mats are a well-liked option because of their superior durability and support.

3. **Resistance Bands**

Resistance bands are adaptable equipment that make your Pilates exercises more difficult. They are often color-coded from light to heavy and available in different resistance levels. Loop resistance bands or long resistance bands with handles work very well for Wall Pilates.

4. **Foam Roller**

Using a foam roller helps promote muscle repair after workouts. In Wall Pilates exercises, it can be utilized to improve strength, flexibility, and balance. To offer sufficient support without being overly rigid, choose a foam roller with a medium density.

5. **Pilates Ball**

A tiny Pilates ball, sometimes referred to as a mini stability ball, gives your workouts an element of instability and encourages deeper activation of your core muscles. These balls may be readily inflated and deflated for transportation. Their diameter is usually between 9 and 12 inches.

6. **Yoga Blocks**

During several Pilates movements, yoga blocks can help to maintain proper posture and provide support. They are quite helpful for novices or people with low range of motion. Blocks composed of high-density foam or cork are sturdy and provide a firm foundation.

7. **Pilates Ring**

A Pilates ring, often called a magic circle, is a flexible ring that is used to increase resistance in a variety of exercises. Muscles in the arms, chest, and inner thighs are especially those that it helps to tone and strengthen. Seek for a ring with padded handles that are cozy.

8. **Towel or Blanket**

There are several uses for a blanket or towel during a Wall Pilates session. It can be used for stretches, to add additional padding to your back or knees, or even as a support to help with certain activities.

Alternatives and DIY Options

It costs very little to practice wall Pilates. Here are some low-cost substitutes and do-it-yourself projects for every necessary item of gear:

1. **Wall Space**

In almost every home, there is a wall. Make sure it's solid and unobstructed by ornaments. Consider outlining your workout space using painter's tape if you're worried about leaving marks on the wall.

2. **Exercise Mat**

For many fitness centers and gyms, the first step into Pilates is mat work. Ironically, Joseph created the tools that participants required to hone their strength and accuracy in order to master the mat activity. The best way to learn mat work is to use the tools as building blocks, where the body is securely supported against gravity.

If you don't have a dedicated exercise mat, alternatives include:

- Towels: To make a padded surface, layer several large towels together.
- Rugs: As an alternative, use a thick, non-slip carpet or rug.
- Blankets: To get the appropriate thickness, fold and stack blankets.

3. **Resistance Bands**

In the absence of resistance bands, consider:

- Old pairs of tights or leggings might offer a comparable degree of resistance.
- Used inner tubes: Resistance bands can be made out of bicycle inner tubes.
- Make Your Own Bands: Use leftover stretchy fabric or cut strips of elastic.

4. **Foam Roller**

For a makeshift foam roller:

- PVC Pipe: To soften the surface of a piece of PVC pipe, wrap it in a towel or yoga mat.
- Rolling Pin: In place of several workouts, you can use a robust rolling pin.
- Pool Noodle: A lightweight substitute is a pool noodle.

5. **Pilates Ball**

If you don't have a Pilates ball:

- Beach Ball: The instability of a Pilates ball can be replicated by a slightly inflated beach ball.
- Cushion: Make use of a tiny, sturdy pillow or cushion.

- Balloon: To get a similar effect, inflate a little balloon.

6. **Yoga Blocks**

For yoga block alternatives:

- Books: Use tape to hold together a stack of hardback books at the appropriate height.
- Bricks: Well-maintained bricks can offer a solid foundation.
- Shoeboxes: To provide stability and weight, stuff shoeboxes with rice or sand.

7. **Pilates Ring**

Substitute a Pilates ring with:

- Belt or Strap: To generate resistance, loop a belt or strap and hold it taut.
- ancient Steering Wheel: An ancient steering wheel might offer resistance and a comparable form.
- Thick Rope: To create a resistance ring, knot a thick rope into a circle.

8. **Towel or Blanket**

Common household items can replace a towel or blanket:

- more Towels: To generate the appropriate support, roll up more towels.
- Scarves: For support and stretching, wear thick scarves.
- Fold old bed linens to provide support and padding.

Tips for Using Alternatives and DIY Equipment

1. **Safety First**

When using alternative or do-it-yourself equipment, safety should always come first. To avoid mishaps, make sure replacements are sturdy and safe. Verify, for instance, that an improvised yoga block or a stack of books won't slip while being used.

2. **Test Before Use**

Make sure alternatives offer the support and resistance you need by testing them before introducing them into your routine. For example, examine the stiffness of a homemade foam roller or the flexibility of an old inner tube.

3. **Adjust as Needed**

If you use different equipment for your exercises, be prepared to make some modest adjustments. Adjust your motions accordingly to maintain proper form and alignment, as the dimensions and resistance of DIY choices may differ from that of regular equipment.

4. **Get Creative**

Be imaginative when coming up with do-it-yourself fixes. Wall Pilates might be properly performed with a lot of commonplace materials. Try out various combinations and materials to see what suits you the best.

Wall Pilates is a minimally equipment-required, versatile, and accessible exercise method. Although professional Pilates equipment can improve your practice, there are several low-cost and do-it-yourself choices accessible. The most important thing is to make sure that the equipment you use safely supports your body and enables you to carry out the activities as intended.

You may get the financial and health benefits of Wall Pilates without going broke with a little ingenuity and resourcefulness. The most crucial thing is to continue practicing consistently and pay attention to your body, regardless of whether you're using a substantial wall, a few common objects, or handcrafted alternatives.

Knowing what you need and looking at other options will prepare you for beginning or continuing your Wall Pilates journey. Recall that the main objective is to improve your physical and mental health, and no matter what tools you employ, you can do this with the appropriate strategy.

Advantages of Pilates in Pregnancy

Pilates strengthens your tummy, back and pelvic floor muscles without straining other joints, so it's a great exercise to do when you're pregnant. Some research suggests that doing Pilates regularly can be as effective as doing pelvic floor exercises.

The main benefit of Pilates is that it targets the exact muscles and functions that can be a problem during pregnancy and after birth, in a safe way.

A stronger transverse abdominus to prevent diastasis recti

At about 20 weeks and often sooner for a second pregnancy, the rectus abdominus will begin to separate along the linea Alba with the two rectus halves moving laterally. This is called diastasis recti. This is a normal occurrence during pregnancy, and this will occur in almost all women. However, when the diastasis recti occurs, there is less support for the lower back, which often results in an increase in low back pain or other discomforts. In addition, women who do not control the size of the diastasis may have difficulty closing it postpartum and may be at risk for an umbilical hernia, especially if there is a subsequent pregnancy without proper closure of the separation.

One of the major misconceptions in existence is usually that women should not work their abdominals while pregnant. It's just a matter of "how" they are working their abdominals. Women should really focus in on the Transverse Abdominis during pregnancy and not on the Rectus or what people see as the six-pack muscles. This means forgoing any ab work involving lifting or holding the torso up against gravity, which would incorporate any of the series of 5, roll ups, or ½ rollbacks or C curve exercises. Instead women should opt for isometric abdominal contractions of the Tranverse, which is like lacing up an internal corset. Strengthening the Transverse will help combat an exaggerated Diastisis Recti, which is something that every mom-to-be should be aware of.

As the abdominals stretch, a small separation will occur between the 2 sides of the Rectus, which are the most superficial layer of the abdominal wall. This is a natural protection response preventing Rectus from having to stretch too far, but if not handled with care, this separation can become over exaggerated and even sometimes not return to its natural state after delivery. This is the number one reason to maintain a strong connection to the deep abdominal muscles, whose job is to keep everything together, even in the stretched state of pregnancy.

It also strengthens the belly muscles, which equip your body far better to cope with the strains caused by the weight of your growing baby. Hormones make the tissues (ligaments) that connect the bones more pliable in pregnancy, making you more prone to injuries.

Stronger pelvic floor muscles

Most women have heard of "Kegel Exercises", but don't really understand the importance the Pelvic Floor during pregnancy. One of the main functions of the pelvic floor is to support the organs in the lower abdominal cavity. As the uterus grows it relies on the pelvic floor more and more for support, which is why it needs to be strengthened. On the flip side, in order to give birth, the Pelvic Floor must completely relax to allow the baby to pass through. Pilates helps women not only feel the contraction of the Pelvic Floor muscles but also the release, ensuring that it is both strong and flexible. It will help to support your bowel, bladder and uterus (womb) as your baby grows and moves down. This may prevent you from leaking small amounts of wee when you cough or sneeze.

A strong Pelvic Floor will also help the body return to its pre pregnancy state more quickly and prevents incontinence.

Improved breath control

Pilates' workout enhances relaxation and controls your breathing, which is important for pregnancy and labor. As the baby grows, the diaphragm is compressed up into the chest, and even though a woman's lung capacity remains the same, it can feel increasingly harder to breathe. Pilates breathing taps into the intercostals muscles lining the ribcage, which allows moms to still feel able to take deep breaths. Pilates breathing also helps keep the thoracic spine (middle back) flexible, which can get very tight during pregnancy. Also, since each exercise in Pilates is associated with the breath connection it makes using the breath during labor much more accessible.

Less discomfort due to muscle & skeletal imbalances

As the baby grows the body does not have any choice but to adapt to make room. This naturally means that posture and alignment will be compromised. While Pilates cannot stop this from happening, it contributes greatly to strengthen the stabilizing muscles, especially those surrounding the hips and pelvis to ensure less discomfort (especially in the low back) as the baby grows and also help with balance issues. Strengthening these muscles also helps to ensure there are no enduring imbalances postpartum.

A quicker recovery & return to pre-pregnancy body

If women lose the connection to their abdominals as they stretch during pregnancy, it will be that much harder to reconnect once the baby is out. It's not just about abs either. So much of being a mom involves lifting, bending over and time spent rounded forward (feeding, changing, pushing a stroller, etc) so strong arms and back are also important to prevent permanent tension, imbalances and bad habits.

Exercises to Avoid During Pregnancy

Pilates' instructors working with pregnant women need to pay careful attention to making sure the chosen exercises are appropriate for this group. Exercises that make the diastasis worse are any movements that require the rectus abdominus to contract strongly against gravity. When the rectus is asked to contract strongly, if the integrity of the muscle is lost, the two halves of the muscle will shorten and contract as two separate units with each half moving laterally. This, in turn, opens the separation further. Precautions need to be taken during any supine exercises that involve lifting the head and shoulders off the ground or lifting both lower extremities off the ground, as well as during plank or push-up positions.

This indicates that most of the traditional abdominal exercises in the Pilates repertoire will not likely be appropriate and may be potentially dangerous with respect to opening the diastasis. Therefore, the Pilates trainer must be proficient in the ability to modify the program and knowledgeable about safe choices for pregnancy. It is also valuable for Pilates' instructors to have knowledge in how to palpate a diastasis so they can screen clients who might be vulnerable to abdominal muscle issue.

Secure & Sound Pregnancy Training

Safe abdominal strengthening during pregnancy should look deeper than the rectus and focus on training of the internal obliques and the transversusabdominus (TVA). Training of the TVA is particularly beneficial because contraction of the TVA directly supports the uterus, and a well toned TVA will help keep the rectus halves closer together and prevent the diastasis from opening excessively. Therefore, TVA training can reduce the size of the diastasis. In addition, training the TVA also helps women prepare for delivery, as one of the roles of this muscle is to assist during forceful expiration (i.e. pushing).

Training of these muscles can occur in all positions, but pregnant women are often most comfortable in sitting and quadruped positions, especially as the pregnancy progresses.

Gentle supine abdominal exercises—such as knee folds, heel slides, pelvic tilts and head lifts—are acceptable and are often much more challenging than one would expect as the abdominal muscles are becoming increasingly weakened.

Tips for modifying Pilates whilst pregnant

Focus on good posture and alignment. At the root of Pilates is the idea of total body integration; moving the entire body as a symphony. This is what a woman has to do during labor and delivery.

The objective of prenatal Pilates is to strengthen instead of stretch out, as joints are susceptible to instability. Don't go to the end range of the joints, as your body won't be able to support that type of movement.

From the second trimester on, many doctors do not advise any supine lying, as it can reduce the supply of blood to a mother's brain. If you do have approval to lie on your back, don't do it for very long. You can also modify exercises by doing them from a seated position, standing, kneeling or lying back propped up on your elbows.

Squats are one of the best ways to open the pelvic outlet. Start working on them in the second trimester when you still have most of your strength — getting up from a squatting position can prove challenging.

Chapter 4: Basic Wall Pilates Exercises

The following exercises are made easy to help you learn and familiarize with Pilates mat exercises. These exercises will help you achieve a strong core together with a stable and flexible body. You can do this on your own or if you choose to enroll under a class, have your instructor teach them to you according to your pace.

Warm-Up Exercises

The warm-up phase is an essential component of practically every other type of physical activity. Regarding Pilates, it is an indispensable component in the process of instructing the fundamentals of the method. As a result, the body is better prepared for subsequent actions, ensuring that it is safe to perform motions that are more difficult. Before beginning an exercise routine, it is important to complete a thorough warm-up. This will assist to raise the temperature of the body and the blood, make the blood vessels more pliable, facilitate a more effective cooling process, enhance the range of motion, and mentally prepare the individual for the subsequent activities.

Stretching, running, simple calisthenics, and flexibility exercises are some examples of the kind of activities that can be included in a straightforward and conventional warm-up. The twist warm-up exercise is a good example of a regimen that you might try out. Initially, locate a location where you are able to perform multiple strides. Skipping is a great way to begin your warm-up sequence. Increase the intensity, range of motion, and twists gradually throughout each set. When you want to take your warm-up to the next level, you could try adding arm swings, torso twists, and even driving your knees a little bit higher. Make certain that your movements are quick and in control at all times. As long as you steadily increase the intensity of the exercise, the number of strides that you choose to perform is entirely up to you.

The Hundred

When it comes to Pilates mat work, this is a traditional exercise. Whenever you enroll in a Pilates class, you will typically be requested to perform this activity at the beginning of the class. While you are warming up the lungs and the abdominal muscles, it is necessary for you to coordinate your movements and breathe simultaneously. Even though it could be difficult, there are alterations that can be made, and if you are able to take control of the situation, you will be able to realize the many advantages that it can provide.

First, you will need to lie on your back with your legs bent in a tabletop position in order to perform the hundred. Check to see that your shins and ankles are aligned in a parallel position to the ground. It is necessary for you to take a breath in here. After that, exhale as you raise your head while maintaining a downward position of your chin.

As you curl your upper spine up to the base of your shoulder blades, you should be using the muscles in your abdominal region. Scoop the abdominal muscles, maintain this position, and then take another breath in. While you are doing this, stretch both your arms and your legs. At this point, exhale and bring your legs in accordance with what you are able to maintain. Raise your arms to a height that is only a few inches above the ground. Maintain your position and catch your breath for a moment. Continue the cycle a number of times, and make sure you don't forget to breathe..

Chest Lift

Initially, this movement could appear to be the same as the abdominal crunch; however, it is essential to keep in mind that the two workouts are distinct abdominal exercises. In order to achieve a flat abdomen region, the chest lift is performed with the intention of bringing the abdominal muscles closer to the mat, so creating a deeper curve.

The first step in accomplishing this is to lie on your back with your knees bent, your legs parallel (with the knee, hip, and ankle all in the same line), and your feet planted firmly on the ground. The next step is to bring your hands behind your head and allow your fingertips to touch. While doing so, keep your shoulders down. Take a few deep breaths and examine your body to ensure that it is standing in a comfortable and balanced position from side to side. At the same time as you are exhaling, bring your stomach closer to your spine and allow it to extend. Move your chin down slightly and slowly elevate your upper spine off the mat until the base of your scapula is just touching it. This will allow you to perform the pose. When you inhale, draw the abdominal muscles deeper. As you lower yourself down the mat, exhale and make sure to keep your abdominal muscles closed. In order to return to a neutral spine position, release the position. Repeat this over and over again, and make sure you don't forget to breathe.

Roll-Up

One of the Pilates mat-work exercises, commonly known as one of the Pilates flat abs exercises, this movement is also considered to be one of the classic Pilates exercises. The abdominal muscles are put under a significant amount of stress, and it is believed to be equivalent to six ordinary sit-ups.

First, you will need to lie down on the floor with your legs straight in order to perform the roll-up. Your shoulders should be relaxed and your tummy should be allowed to descend toward the floor. Make sure that your shoulders are not touching your ears. Take a few deep breaths and check your alignment as you do so. Ensure that your ribs are positioned in a downward position and that your scapula is firmly rooted in your back. Ensure that your fingertips are pointed in the direction of the wall behind you by positioning your arms so that they are raised over your head and back. First, take a deep breath in, then lift your arms up over your head while keeping your scapula down. In order to join the action, you should allow your chin to drop and twist your head and upper spine in the same direction. As you continue to curl your body "up and over" in a smooth motion toward your toes, exhale and perform the exercise. When you breathe in and out, you should make an effort to pull your abdominal muscles in and deepen the curve of your spine. As you reach for your toes, be sure that your head is tucked in, that your back is rounded, and that your abdominal muscles are deep. While you are attempting to pull the lower abdominal muscles in, take a deep breath in and then bring it all the way into your back and pelvis. After then, bring your tail bone under your body and start uncurling your spine vertebrae by vertebrae until you are back on the floor.

Rolling Like a Ball

The Pilates mat-work activity that is considered to be the most traditional is almost always included in a Pilates class. There are some individuals who are able to wrap up like a pill bug with ease and have a great deal of success while you are doing so. Those individuals, on the other hand, who have low backs and find it difficult to round their backs may initially find this exercise to be somewhat demanding. In addition to helping to strengthen the abdominal muscles and stimulate the spine, this action also helps to tune the flow of our body's movement and breathing.

First things first, you need to make sure that you are sitting on your mat completely and that your hands are clasped over your shins somewhere just above your ankles. The next step is to relax your shoulders and make your back wider. Moreover, you should deepen your abdominal muscles and create a wonderful curvature in your spine. Considering that your neck is a component of that long curve, you should avoid tucking your head. The following step is to lift your feet off the mat and balance on your sit bones. This is the next set of instructions. Take a deep breath in as you draw your lower abdominal muscles in and up to begin yourself going, and then take another deep breath as you attempt to roll back. Keep in mind that you should only roll as far as your shoulders and not onto your neck. Maintain a scooping position with your spine curled while you exhale. To return to an upright position when you breath, use your abdominal muscles. You should maintain your equilibrium while performing this movement, and you should do it multiple times. Additionally, you should not forget to breathe.

One-Leg Circle

When it comes to evaluating one's core strength, this exercise is the most effective. In order to accomplish this, the abdominal muscle should exert a great deal of effort in order to maintain the stability of the pelvis and shoulders throughout the entire movement. It is a focal exercise, and all of the Pilates principles can be seen present in this movement to a significant degree.

For the purpose of getting ready, you should lie down on your back with your arms at your sides and your rear legs extended on the floor. Get in touch with your body and make sure that the weight of your shoulders and hips on each side is balanced. Begin by drawing your abdominal muscles in toward your spine and securing your shoulders and pelvis. Then, without rising your hip, stretch one leg toward the sky and lengthen it. Do this without lifting your hip. However, you should make sure that your hips are sturdy and firmly planted on the mat. You could wish to bend your knee slightly here and there. Taking a deep breath, cross the leg that is stretched to the hip of the opposing side. As you lower it a few inches, exhale as you do so. Open the leg outside and sweep it around in a circular pattern back to the center while maintaining control of the movement. Make a number of rounds in each direction, and as you are doing so, take deep breaths and exhale slowly.

Open Leg Balance

In addition, this movement is among the most effective exercises for evaluating the strength of the lower abdominals and the core. It is highly likely that you will lose your balance while holding this position if you have a weak core. In addition, you will be able to stretch your legs and your back by extending and stretching your back while you are in this pose.

When you begin to perform the stance, you should begin by sitting down. Make an effort to move your feet closer to your torso while maintaining an open knee position and bringing your feet together. You should position your arms such that they are inside your legs and grab your ankles while maintaining a lowered posture with your shoulders. As you continue to extend one leg after the other, the next step is to pull in the abdominal muscles and pay attention to elevating the lower abdominal muscles. Attempt to maintain your balance and hold the stance for at least five counts. Take charge of the situation and fold one leg after the other in a methodical and controlled manner, bringing each leg down.

Plank Pose

One of the most well-known exercises, the plank is also utilized in a variety of other wellness practices. In order to develop a strong core and a sturdy frame, it is a popular technique that involves challenging the entire body. Although the plank may appear to be similar to a standard push-up, the difference is that rather than moving up and down, you remain in a higher posture with your shoulders extended.

Start by getting down on your knees and bringing both hands in front of you with your fingers firmly planted on the ground. This is the plank position. Your abdominal muscles should be engaged, and your spine should be lengthened as you lean forward and bring your shoulders into alignment with your wrists. Next, progressively extend your legs straight while maintaining a close proximity between them. Maintaining the stance while taking deep breaths and allowing the air to expand into your back and lower ribs is your goal.

The Side Kick Series

It is beneficial to develop and tone the muscles of the hips, abdominal region, and thighs by performing the exercises that are included in this series. They make an effort to place an emphasis on length and make use of the powerhouse to stabilize the trunk through the movement of the lower body.

Laying on your side with your shoulders, hips, knees, ankles, and ears aligned is the first step in the setup process. You should lift your ribs away from the mat in order to maintain the alignment of your neck and back. It is recommended that the leading hand be placed on the mat in front of the chest. It is possible to use this to assist stabilize you, but you should not rely on it too heavily. In order to improve your balance, you should then move your legs forward slightly. While maintaining a Pilates posture, rotate the legs gently.

Kick Front

This can be accomplished by first lifting the top leg a few inches and then flexing the foot. After that, bring the upper leg as far forward as possible and attempt to perform a pulse kick while your kick is at its full length.

a) Take a Step Backward

You should point your toe and move your leg to the back while maintaining the length of your leg simultaneously. Make sure that you do not shift the pelvis and that you remain in this posture for a length of time. Reach as far as you possibly can. The next step is to flex your foot and kick once again in the direction of the front.

b) Leg Lifts to the Side

Take a deep breath in as you stretch your entire body from head to toe. Breathe out while you utilize your abdominal muscles to lift both of your legs a few inches above the surface of the mat. Try to keep your inner thoughts organized. As you bring your legs closer to the mat, take a deep breath and stretch them.

c) Moving Your Feet Up and Down

Additionally, from the position in which you have set up, make sure that your abdominal muscles are pulled in and stretched upward. As you kick your upper leg toward the ceiling, you should then stretch the top leg. During this process, it is essential to ensure that the pelvis does not tilt backward and that the hipbones continue to remain stacked. To go down, push your abdominal muscles up against the lengthening of your leg. This will allow you to move down.

The Mermaid Side Stretch

By holding this pose, you will be able to open up the sides of your body and extend the muscles that control your motions. You can incorporate it into your routine as a moderate warm-up exercise or as a more vigorous activity. Both of these uses are possible.

Begin by sitting on the floor with both of your legs folded to the left side. This will prepare you for the mermaid stretch technique. While maintaining an erect position, place the right hand on the floor in a flat position to give support. As you attempt to raise the arm above the head, be sure that the opposite shoulder is positioned so that it is not touching your left ear.

Keep your hips firmly planted on the ground while you lengthen and extend to the side. Extend your spine to its furthest extent and then turn it to the opposite side. Take care not to allow your ribs to protrude forward while you are doing this. To achieve a greater stretch, move the hand that is providing support further. In order to make the exercise more challenging, you can even fold the support elbow. To come back, raise your torso up by using your abdominal muscles.

Make sure to bring the left arm down this time and use it as a support so that you may stretch on the other side. The right arm should be extended and the reach should be as far as possible without compromising the integrity of the shoulder. When you have finished taking a few breaths, return to the beginning posture by using your core.

Single Leg Stretch

This technique is designed to train the abdominal muscles to move and begin from the center of the body. Additionally, it assists in the development of a robust support and works to stabilize the trunk when the limbs are in motion.

Laying on your back with your knees bent and your shins parallel to the floor is the first step in getting ready. Exhale and inhale while you are in this position. The next step is to pull your abdominal muscles and curl your shoulders and head all the way up to the points of your chest. As you continue to do this, your left leg should be extended at a 45-degree angle. The opposite leg should remain in the initial position, and the right hand should be used to grab holding of the right ankle. Additionally, transition the left hand to the right knee while keeping the upper body curvature throughout the entire movement. Turn your body so that your left hand is now on your left ankle and your right hand is on your left knee. This time, switch your legs. In the event that you are already experiencing a great deal of strain in your neck and shoulders, the legs should be switched numerous times and then released.

Spine Stretch

When it comes to strengthening the hamstrings and the back muscles, the spine stretch is an excellent workout. Because it helps you get ready for more difficult activities, it is effective in practically any kind of workout you can give yourself.

To begin, assume a tall seated position with your legs stretched out shoulder-width apart. As you inhale, bring both of your arms forward until they are at shoulder height. By exhaling, you should make an effort to stretch your spine and curve forward till you reach your toes. As you take a deep breath in, extend your reach as far as you possibly can. Take a deep breath out and then use your lower abdominal muscles to return to the starting posture.

Double Leg Stretch

The double leg stretch is an excellent abdominal exercise that targets the powerhouse and requires a great deal of endurance from the core by drawing strength from the powerhouse.

The initial step in performing this workout is to curl up. Assume a supine position with your shins horizontal to the ground. While you are holding your ankles or shins, pull your abdominal muscles in and curve your upper body slightly. Stretch your limbs out in opposing directions and reach as far as you can. Maintain a taut abdominal contraction and keep your lower back firmly planted on the mat. Pull yourself back into the middle, and then coil up once again. Your chest and head should remain raised, and you should avoid lowering the curvature. It is important to remember to keep yourself aligned to the center when you perform the extension and pulling back to the center multiple times.

The Saw

In order to stretch the back and the hamstrings, the saw was invented. As you become more familiar with it, it becomes extremely intriguing as you deal with the oppositional dynamic between your various body parts. It is a good method to experience opposition stretch, and as you begin to appreciate it, it becomes really exciting.

You should begin by sitting up straight on your sit bones and extending both of your legs in front of you. Extend your arms to the side until they are perpendicular to your shoulders. Take a deep breath in as you rotate your entire torso while maintaining a steady hip position. When you follow your back hand and turn your upper torso as if you were curling yourself, exhale as you do so simultaneously. At the same time as you are attempting to reach the fingers of one hand across the other foot, stretch. Maintain the position until you are able to extend as far as you possibly can, and then take a deep breath before returning to a seated position. Carry out the workout on both sides, and be sure to remember to maintain your breathing throughout the process.

The Swan

After performing a significant number of forward flexions, the swan is called an extension exercise because it is designed to assist you in counter stretching. In addition to opening up the front of the body, it also provides the chest and the belly with a considerable amount of expansion and flexibility. As an additional benefit, it helps to strengthen the abdominal region, as well as the shoulders, back, thighs, pelvis, glutes, and hamstrings.

In order to perform this posture, you will need to lie on your mat with your back bent and your arms close to your body. The next step is to bring your hands under your shoulders and make sure they are not in contact with your ears. This can be accomplished by bending your elbows. In addition to that, make sure to keep the legs together. The next step is to contract the muscles in your abdominal region. develop a long upward arc in the upper portion of your body by inhaling as you stretch your spine and press your forearms and hands into the mat. This will help you develop a long posture. While you continue to elevate the abdominal muscles, exhale. Your spine should be lengthened, and you should slowly return to the mat after releasing the arc. It is necessary to repeat this sequence multiple times.

Pilates Push-up

There is a more sophisticated form of the push-up that is called the Pilates push-up. When it comes to improving the core and arms, it is highly beneficial. Additionally, it is the most effective method for training endurance, strength, and stability.

To begin, assume the standing position while maintaining the appropriate posture for Pilates. Raise your arms over your head in a straight formation. When you are attempting to place your hands on the mat, bend your body outward. Place yourself in a plank position and make sure that your shoulders are not touching your ears when you leave the position. The next step is to take a little break while maintaining the front plank position. This will assist in stabilizing your shoulders. Proceed to lower yourself toward the mat, exactly as you would when performing a standard push-up. Assume a plank stance, walk backwards, and then roll up to a standing position once more.

Chapter 5: Intermediate Wall Pilates Exercises

By introducing resistance and support into your Pilates program through the utilization of wall Pilates exercises, you may make your routine more complex and interesting. In addition to providing you with stability, these workouts will test your core strength and present you with a challenge. Within the realm of Wall Pilates, the Wall Plank, the Wall Bridge, and the Wall Push-Ups are three exercises that are considered to be of an intermediate level of difficulty. This chapter will concentrate on these three exercises. Every single workout comes with a detailed guide to the method, as well as an explanation of the benefits of using the technique.

Wall Plank

Technique

The Wall Plank is a modified variation of the standard plank exercise that involves using the wall as a support when performing the exercise. The abdominal muscles, shoulders, and arms are the primary targets of this workout.

1. To get started, you should arrange yourself such that you are facing the wall and that you are around an arm's length away from touching it. Place both of your hands on the wall at a height that is equivalent to your shoulders and at a distance that is wide enough to accommodate your shoulders. In order to get the desired effect, it is essential that your fingers are pointing upwards and that your arms are fully extended above your head.

2. To ensure that your body is in a straight line from your head to your heels, move your feet backwards until you reach this position. You ought to posture your body in this manner whenever possible. Your weight should be distributed evenly between your hands and feet, and the wall should be positioned at a little angle to your torso. It is recommended that your body be positioned in this manner.

3. Engage your core and strengthen the muscles in your abdominal region to prevent your hips from sagging or lifting. This will help you avoid unnecessary discomfort. It is imperative that you maintain a straight line with your body at all times.

4. The objective of this workout is to keep your body in this position for around thirty to sixty seconds while focusing on your breathing. Ensure that your core remains engaged throughout the entire process of breathing in through your nose and out through your mouth. Both of these breathing patterns are important.

5. After carefully walking your feet back towards the wall, you will be able to return to the beginning position. After that, you will stand up straight. When you do this, you will be brought back to the point where you began.

Benefits

- When performed correctly, the Wall Plank is an excellent exercise for strengthening the abdominal muscles, particularly the transverse abdominis and the obliques. Core strength is achieved by this exercise.

- In addition to enhancing the strength of the shoulder, the isometric hold is also responsible for contributing to the improvement of shoulder stability.

- One of the benefits of this exercise is that it helps improve posture by working the muscles that are placed around the spine.

- This exercise provides a low-impact alternative to the standard plank, which in turn decreases the amount of pressure that is imposed on the wrists and lower back as a result of the exercise.

Wall Bridge

Technique

For a terrific workout that targets the glutes, hamstrings, and lower back while also making use of the wall for additional resistance and support, the Wall Bridge is an excellent opportunity.

1. At the beginning of the exercise, you should lie on your back with your feet planted on the wall and your knees bent at a right angle of ninety degrees. This is the starting position. With your palms facing down, your arms should be lying at your sides, and the distance between your feet should be equal to the width of your hips.

2. You will need to activate your core muscles as well as your glutes in order to get ready for the workout. Put pressure on your glutes and tighten the muscles in your abdominal region.

3. By applying pressure via your feet and pushing your hips toward the ceiling, you can create an elevated hip position. Consequently, this will result in a line that is straight from your shoulders to your knees. It is imperative that you check that your hips do not arch or sag in any part.

4. Continue to Hold the Position: Hold this bridge position for a few seconds while maintaining the tightness in your glutes and keeping your core engaged. This will help you maintain the position.

5. a drop While you are slowly lowering your hips back to the starting position, it is important to make sure that you are controlling the process with your core and glutes exercises.

6. It is recommended that you execute ten to fifteen repetitions as part of a single set.

Benefits

- Glute Activation: The Wall Bridge is an efficient exercise that targets and strengthens the gluteal muscles, which are crucial for improved strength throughout the lower body. This exercise is also known as the muscular activation exercise.

- In addition to this, it works the hamstrings, which leads to an increase in the tone of the muscles as well as an increase in their flexibility.

- Providing Support for the Lower Back: Participating in exercises that strengthen the muscles of the lower back can assist in reducing the discomfort experienced in the back and improving the stability of the spine.

- The term "pelvic stability exercises" refers to a group of exercises that improve pelvic stability and assist in the correction of conditions that are associated with irregular pelvic tilt.

Wall Push-Ups

Technique

Push-ups on the wall are a modified version of the conventional push-up that are designed to make them more accessible while still providing a challenging workout for the upper body. Wall push-ups are a modification of the standard push-up.

1. To get started, you should arrange yourself such that you are facing the wall and that you are around an arm's length away from touching it. When you are in a comfortable posture, place your hands on the wall at shoulder height and shoulder-width apart. Your fingers should be directed upwards.

2. Simply walking your feet backwards slightly can allow you to arrange your body at an angle. Because of this, your body will be positioned at an angle. From your head to your heels, you should form a straight line, and the distance between your feet should be equal to the width of your hips. Maintain this position for the entire exercise.

3. The elbows of your lower body should be bent, and you should gradually lower your chest toward the wall while keeping a straight line around your body. This should be done while maintaining a straight line around your body. Position your elbows so that they are at a 45-degree angle to your torso. Place your elbows in this position.

4. When performing the push back exercise, you should press through your hands in order to straighten your arms and return to the beginning posture. Make sure that your core is engaged at all times so that you can keep your body from becoming unstable.

5. It is recommended that you execute ten to fifteen repetitions as part of a single set.

Benefits

- Upper Body Strength: Wall Push-Ups are an excellent exercise for improving upper body strength since they target the chest, shoulders, and triceps.

- Engagement of the Core: This exercise also utilizes the core muscles because it requires the participant to maintain a straight body line.

- Improved Stability Thanks to the wall's ability to provide support, this exercise is an excellent choice for novices who are looking to build their confidence before moving on to floor push-ups.

- Joint-Friendly: Because this alteration eliminates the strain that is placed on the shoulders and wrists, it is appropriate for individuals who have problems with their joints.

Chapter 6: Advanced Wall Pilates Exercises

For individuals who are prepared to take their Pilates practice to the next level from the very beginning, advanced wall Pilates exercises offer a progression that is not only challenging but also rewarding. During the course of this chapter, we are going to discuss three more advanced exercises. These activities are the Wall Pike, the Wall Scissors, and the Wall Handstand Preparation. Each and every one of the exercises comes with a detailed set of instructions as well as a description of the benefits that may be gained from doing them.

Wall Pike

Technique

The Wall Pike is a demanding exercise that enhances core strength, shoulder stability, and flexibility.

1. Take a plank position with your feet pressed against the wall and your hands positioned shoulder-width apart on the floor. This is the starting position for the exercise. The starting position is in this position. From your head to your heels, it is essential that your body is in a straight line all the way down to your feet.

2. While doing so, contract the muscles in your abdominal region and begin to elevate your hips toward the sky. This will help you activate your core and lift your hips. Walk your feet up the wall while you are lifting, being sure to keep your legs in a straight position.

3. Continue to lift your hips until your body forms an inverted V shape, with your torso and legs straight. This is the Pike position. Your ability to manufacture a pike will be enabled by this. Ensure that your head is facing your feet and that it is positioned between your arms in the correct posture.

4. Carry on with it Continue to Hold the Position: Hold the pike position for a few seconds while concentrating on maintaining the position. Make sure that your legs are straight and that your core is strong.

5. After you have returned to the starting position, carefully lower your hips to the plank position while walk your feet down the wall in a controlled manner. This should be done as you are performing the exercise.

6. There should be between five and 10 repetitions of the exercise performed for one set.

Benefits

- To increase core strength, the Wall Pike is a fantastic exercise since it strengthens the abdominal muscles, particularly the lower abdominal muscles. This makes it an excellent choice for increasing core strength.

- Shoulder Stability: Because it is performed in a weight-bearing position, it helps to increase the stability and strength of the shoulders.

- The hamstrings and shoulders are the primary muscles that are worked during this exercise, which aims to improve physical flexibility.

- A Workout That Targets the Entire Body: In order to provide a comprehensive workout, this exercise targets a wide variety of muscle groups, including the abdominal muscles, the shoulders, and the legs for example.

Wall Scissors

Technique

Wall Scissors is an advanced exercise that challenges your core, leg strength, and coordination.

1. Position yourself so that you are lying on your back with your legs extended up the wall. Your body should be at a right angle to the wall. The starting position is in this position. I would suggest that you rest your arms by your sides with your palms facing down. This is the recommended position.

2. Raise your hips off the ground and activate your core by clenching your abdominal muscles and elevating your hips off the ground. This will help build your core strength. The result of this is that your hips will move slightly away from the wall.

3. For the scissor leg exercise, bring one leg down toward the floor while keeping the other leg against the wall. This will allow you to perform the exercise efficiently. It is important that the motion of your legs be controlled and comparable to that of scissors.

4. In order to switch legs, you must first bring the leg that is lowered up to the wall and then bring the other leg down towards the floor to complete the switch. The alternate leg exercise is the name given to this motion. Throughout the entirety of the process, ensure that you keep a smooth and consistent moving motion.

5. Making sure that your core remains engaged during the entirety of your workout is really crucial. Additionally, throughout this period, you need to make sure that your lower back is not making contact with the floor.

6. It is recommended that a total of ten to fifteen repetitions be performed for each leg during the course of one set.

Benefits

- Developing Core Strength: Wall Scissors are an excellent workout for developing core strength since they target the lower abdominal muscles.

- Strengthening of the Leg Muscles and Increased Flexibility in the Legs: This exercise helps to strengthen the leg muscles and increase flexibility in the hip flexors and hamstrings.

- The practice of this exercise, which consists of alternating between different foot movements, is beneficial to both control and coordination.

- Spinal Stability: When you exercise the muscles in your deep core, you aid to contribute to the maintenance of your spine's stability.

6.3 Wall Handstand Preparation

Technique

Wall Handstand Preparation is a powerful exercise for building the strength and confidence needed for full handstands.

1. Your hands should be placed shoulder-width apart on the floor, and your feet should be forced against the wall. This is the starting posture, which is known as the dog stance. The downward dog position is the name given to this particular stance.

2. While you are carefully walking your feet up the wall, you will be moving your body into a position that is more vertical. Walking one's feet up the wall is the name of this particular workout. Let's assume that your hands are securely planted on the ground and that they are spaced shoulder-width apart from one another.

3. A straight line should be established from your hands to your hips once your feet have reached the height of your hips. Adjust your body so that this line is formed. Your body is positioned in this manner presently. In order to achieve the best results, it is recommended that you place your head between your arms and look at the ground below you.

4. You should tense your abdominal muscles and maintain this position for a few seconds while keeping your body in a straight line. Repeat this process several times. The acronym for this particular exercise is "engage core and hold."

5. Walk Your Feet Down: Beginning in the starting position, return to the starting position in a controlled manner by walking your feet down the wall in a slow direction. Perform this exercise in order to complete the exercise.

6. There should be between five and 10 repetitions of the exercise performed for one set.

Benefits

- Strength in the upper body, specifically in the shoulders, arms, and upper back, can be significantly improved with the use of the Wall Handstand Preparation, which is an outstanding method.

- Enhancing Core Stability: This exercise helps to enhance core stability and control, which is one of the most essential components of maintaining balance while completing a handstand.

- This practice helps develop confidence as well as body awareness, both of which are required for beginning to perform complete handstands. Developing confidence is necessary for beginning to perform full handstands.

- This activity helps improve balance and coordination, both of which are needed for advanced Pilates as well as other forms of fitness. The practice of this movement helps improve balance and coordination.

Chapter 7: Beyond Exercise E- book.

Diet Plan

The popular form of exercise known as wall Pilates is a style of Pilates that makes use of a wall as a support, bringing a new and interesting dimension to the standard Pilates workouts. Improved balance, stability, and general muscle activation are all outcomes that can be achieved through the utilization of this strategy. However, in order to get the most out of Wall Pilates, it is necessary to supplement the workouts with a diet that is well-balanced along with the exercises. For the purpose of assisting women in achieving their best possible results, this guide offers thorough dietary advice for Pilates practitioners as well as sample meal plans.

Nutrition Tips for Pilates Practitioners

1. **Balanced Macronutrients:**
   - Proteins are necessary for the growth and repair of lean muscle tissue. Lean meats, fish, eggs, dairy products, legumes, and plant-based proteins such as tofu and tempeh should all be included in your diet.
   - Carbohydrates are a source of energy that is essential for physical activity. Instead of processed sugars and flours, choose complex carbohydrates like whole grains, fruits, and vegetables as your primary source of carbohydrates.
   - Fats: Consuming healthy fats is beneficial to one's general health and helps in the process of absorbing fat-soluble vitamins. Ingredients such as avocados, nuts, seeds, olive oil, and fatty fish are examples of sources.

2. **Hydration:**
   - Keeping yourself hydrated is extremely important because even slight dehydration can have a negative impact on both your physical performance and your cognitive function. Aim to drink at least eight to ten glasses of water every day, and even more if you are sweating significantly while you are working out.

3. **Pre-Workout Nutrition**:

    o   Consuming a light snack 1–2 hours prior to your Wall Pilates session can be beneficial in terms of providing fuel for your workout. Try something that mixes carbohydrates and protein, like a banana with nut butter or a yogurt with berries. Both of these options are great options.

4. **Post-Workout Nutrition**:

    o   Within thirty to sixty minutes of finishing your workout, you should provide your body with a meal or snack that is high in carbohydrates and protein. The muscles are repaired and glycogen levels are restored as a result of this. There are many examples of healthy foods, such as a turkey sandwich on whole grain bread, a quinoa salad with chickpeas, and a smoothie that contains protein powder.

5. **Nutrient Timing**:

    o   By distributing meals and snacks at regular intervals throughout the day, one may help maintain their energy levels and support the recuperation of their muscles. Your daily goal should be to consume three main meals and two to three snacks.

6. **Micronutrients**:

    o   When it comes to general health and performance, vitamins and minerals are absolutely necessary. Make sure that your diet contains a wide range of colored fruits and vegetables so that you may satisfy your requirements for micronutrients. If you have specific deficiencies, you might want to think about taking supplements, but before you do so, you should talk to your healthcare professional.

7. **Listening to Your Body**:

    o   Pay attention to indicators that communicate hunger and fullness. Maintaining a healthy weight and supporting your fitness objectives can be accomplished by eating just when you are hungry and ending when you are full and satisfied.

Sample Meal Plans

During your Wall Pilates sessions, the following three sample meal plans will assist you in guiding your nutrition in the right direction. The primary goal of each plan is to supply you with a balanced supply of macronutrients, important vitamins, and minerals to assist your path toward a healthier lifestyle.

Sample Meal Plan 1

Breakfast:

- Greek yogurt parfait with honey, mixed berries, and a sprinkle of granola.
- A glass of water or herbal tea.

Morning Snack:

- An apple with a handful of almonds.

Lunch:

- Grilled chicken breast with quinoa, mixed greens, cherry tomatoes, cucumbers, and a lemon-tahini dressing.
- A glass of water.

Afternoon Snack:

- Carrot sticks with hummus.

Dinner:

- Baked salmon with a side of brown rice and steamed broccoli.
- Mixed green salad with olive oil and balsamic vinegar dressing.
- A glass of water or herbal tea.

Evening Snack:

- A small bowl of mixed berries.

Sample Meal Plan 2

Breakfast:

- Smoothie made with spinach, banana, protein powder, almond milk, and a tablespoon of flaxseeds.
- A glass of water or green tea.

Morning Snack:

- A piece of whole grain toast with avocado spread and a sprinkle of chia seeds.

Lunch:

- Lentil soup with a side of mixed greens and a whole grain roll.
- A glass of water.

Afternoon Snack:

- A small bowl of mixed nuts and dried fruit.

Dinner:

- Stir-fried tofu with mixed vegetables (bell peppers, snap peas, carrots) served over brown rice.
- A glass of water or herbal tea.

Evening Snack:

- A slice of watermelon or another seasonal fruit.

Sample Meal Plan 3

Breakfast:

- Oatmeal topped with sliced bananas, walnuts, and a drizzle of honey.
- A glass of water or black coffee.

Morning Snack:

- A small pear and a handful of pumpkin seeds.

Lunch:

- Turkey and avocado wrap with whole grain tortilla, spinach, tomatoes, and a light yogurt-based dressing.
- A glass of water.

Afternoon Snack:

- Cottage cheese with pineapple chunks.

Dinner:

- Grilled shrimp with a side of quinoa salad (quinoa, black beans, corn, bell peppers, cilantro, lime juice).
- A glass of water or herbal tea.

Evening Snack:

- A few dark chocolate squares.

Additional Tips for Sustainable Eating Habits

1. **Meal Prep**:
    - Preparing meals in advance can help you stay on track with your nutrition goals. Dedicate a day or two each week to cook and portion out meals and snacks.
2. **Mindful Eating**:
    - Eating slowly and without distractions can enhance your enjoyment of food and help prevent overeating. Focus on the taste, texture, and aroma of your meals.
3. **Portion Control**:
    - Be mindful of portion sizes to avoid consuming excess calories. Use smaller plates and bowls to help manage portions.
4. **Healthy Swaps**:

- Make simple swaps to boost nutrition without sacrificing flavor. For instance, use Greek yogurt instead of sour cream, choose whole grain pasta over regular pasta, and opt for baked instead of fried foods.

5. **Enjoy Treats in Moderation**:
    - It's okay to indulge occasionally. Balance is key to a sustainable diet. Enjoy your favorite treats in moderation without guilt.

By combining a balanced diet with your Wall Pilates workouts, you'll be well on your way to achieving your fitness goals. Remember that consistency is crucial, and making gradual, sustainable changes to your diet and exercise routine will yield the best long-term results. Whether you're a beginner or an experienced Pilates practitioner, these nutrition tips and meal plans can help support your journey to a healthier, stronger you.

Workout Plan

The concepts of classic Pilates can be incorporated into wall Pilates, which is an excellent method to combine the support and stability that a wall provides with the Pilates principles. This technique has the potential to enhance both core strength and flexibility, as well as balance and general body tone. An in-depth guide to constructing an effective Wall Pilates workout plan for women, including a weekly training schedule and progression tactics, is presented here. The manual contains more than a thousand words.

Weekly Workout Schedule

Week 1-2: Foundation and Basics

Objective: To build a strong foundation, familiarize with basic moves, and ensure proper form and alignment.

Monday: Core Focus

- **Warm-up:** Gentle stretches (5 minutes)
- **Wall Roll-Down:** 10 reps

- **Wall Plank:** 3 sets of 20 seconds
- **Wall Bridge:** 3 sets of 10 reps
- **Wall Hundred:** 3 sets of 10 breaths
- **Cool-down:** Light stretching (5 minutes)

Tuesday: Lower Body Strength

- **Warm-up:** Dynamic leg swings (5 minutes)
- **Wall Squats:** 3 sets of 12 reps
- **Wall Lunges:** 3 sets of 10 reps each leg
- **Wall Side Leg Lifts:** 3 sets of 15 reps each leg
- **Wall Heel Raises:** 3 sets of 15 reps
- **Cool-down:** Hamstring and quad stretches (5 minutes)

Wednesday: Rest or Light Activity

- Gentle yoga or a brisk walk (30 minutes)

Thursday: Upper Body and Posture

- **Warm-up:** Arm circles and shoulder rolls (5 minutes)
- **Wall Push-ups:** 3 sets of 12 reps
- **Wall Angel Wings:** 3 sets of 10 reps
- **Wall Shoulder Stretch:** 3 sets of 15 seconds each arm
- **Wall Tricep Dips:** 3 sets of 10 reps
- **Cool-down:** Shoulder and arm stretches (5 minutes)

Friday: Full Body Integration

- **Warm-up:** Full body dynamic stretches (5 minutes)
- **Wall Roll-Down to Plank:** 3 sets of 5 reps
- **Wall Squat with Arm Raises:** 3 sets of 12 reps
- **Wall Leg Circles:** 3 sets of 10 reps each leg
- **Wall Plank with Leg Lift:** 3 sets of 10 reps each leg
- **Cool-down:** Total body stretches (5 minutes)

Saturday: Flexibility and Balance

- **Warm-up:** Gentle stretches (5 minutes)
- **Wall Assisted Standing Split:** 3 sets of 15 seconds each leg
- **Wall Tree Pose:** 3 sets of 20 seconds each leg
- **Wall Forward Bend:** 3 sets of 30 seconds
- **Wall Side Stretch:** 3 sets of 15 seconds each side
- **Cool-down:** Relaxation stretches (5 minutes)

Sunday: Rest or Light Activity

- Light activity such as walking, gentle swimming, or restorative yoga

Week 3-4: Intermediate Moves and Increased Intensity

Objective: To introduce intermediate exercises, increase intensity, and start integrating more complex movements.

Monday: Core and Stability

- **Warm-up:** Gentle core activation (5 minutes)
- **Wall Roll-Down with Twist:** 3 sets of 8 reps each side
- **Wall Plank with Arm Lift:** 3 sets of 10 reps each arm
- **Wall Single Leg Bridge:** 3 sets of 8 reps each leg
- **Wall Side Plank:** 3 sets of 15 seconds each side
- **Cool-down:** Core stretches (5 minutes)

Tuesday: Lower Body Power

- **Warm-up:** Dynamic leg swings and hip circles (5 minutes)
- **Wall Bulgarian Split Squat:** 3 sets of 8 reps each leg
- **Wall Skater Squats:** 3 sets of 10 reps each leg
- **Wall Sumo Squats:** 3 sets of 12 reps
- **Wall Calf Raises with Hold:** 3 sets of 12 reps
- **Cool-down:** Lower body stretches (5 minutes)

Wednesday: Rest or Light Activity

- Gentle stretching or a casual bike ride (30 minutes)

Thursday: Upper Body and Core Integration

- **Warm-up:** Arm swings and shoulder warm-up (5 minutes)
- **Wall Push-ups with Rotation:** 3 sets of 10 reps

- **Wall Angel Wings with Resistance Band:** 3 sets of 12 reps
- **Wall Tricep Dips with Leg Extension:** 3 sets of 8 reps each leg
- **Wall Pike Push-ups:** 3 sets of 8 reps
- **Cool-down:** Arm and shoulder stretches (5 minutes)

Friday: Dynamic Full Body

- **Warm-up:** Full body warm-up (5 minutes)
- **Wall Burpees:** 3 sets of 10 reps
- **Wall Jump Squats:** 3 sets of 12 reps
- **Wall Mountain Climbers:** 3 sets of 20 reps
- **Wall Leg Scissors:** 3 sets of 10 reps each leg
- **Cool-down:** Full body stretches (5 minutes)

Saturday: Enhanced Flexibility and Balance

- **Warm-up:** Gentle mobility work (5 minutes)
- **Wall Assisted Standing Split with Reach:** 3 sets of 20 seconds each leg
- **Wall Dancer Pose:** 3 sets of 15 seconds each leg
- **Wall Forward Fold with Deep Stretch:** 3 sets of 30 seconds
- **Wall Side Bend with Deep Reach:** 3 sets of 20 seconds each side
- **Cool-down:** Relaxation stretches (5 minutes)

Sunday: Rest or Light Activity

- Light activity such as nature walk, light stretching, or meditation

Progression Strategies

1. Increase Repetitions and Sets:

- Start by adding 1-2 reps to each set every week.
- Gradually increase the number of sets from 3 to 4 or even 5, depending on your fitness level.

2. Add Resistance:

- Exercises such as Wall Angel Wings and Wall Squats can be made more challenging by incorporating resistance bands into the workout.
- When performing wall squats or wall lunges, you can further push your muscles by holding light dumbbells in your hands.

3. Enhance the Difficulty of Exercises:

- Start with Wall Push-ups and work your way up to more difficult varieties such as Wall Pike Push-ups or Wall Push-ups with one leg lifted.
- You should begin by performing basic wall planks and then progress to more complex variations such as the wall plank with arm lift or the wall side plank with leg lift.

4. Increase Hold Time for Isometric Exercises:

- For exercises such as the Wall Plank or the Wall Side Plank, progressively increase the amount of time you hold each exercise by five to ten seconds weekly.
- The goal is to hold the Wall Squat position for a longer period of time, gradually increasing the time from twenty seconds to sixty seconds.

5. Integrate More Complex Movements:

- Combine exercises to create compound movements, such as Wall Roll-Down to Plank with a Leg Lift or Wall Lunge with an Arm Raise.

- Add dynamic movements like Wall Jump Squats or Wall Burpees to elevate the heart rate and enhance cardiovascular benefits.

6. Focus on Form and Mind-Body Connection:

- Put in consistent effort to improve your form in order to reduce the risk of injury and get the most of the benefits that each exercise provides.
- It is important to pay attention to your breathing and make sure that you are breathing in a deep and rhythmic manner in order to support your movements and activate your core.

7. Track Progress and Set Goals:

- Remember to keep a workout journal in which you record your repetitions, sets, and any modifications to your regimen.
- Set short-term goals that are attainable, such as increasing the amount of time you hold the exercise or adding resistance, and long-term goals, such as becoming proficient in more complex exercises.

8. Listen to Your Body:

- Pay close attention to how your body reacts when you raise the volume and intensity of your workout.
- Ensure that you give yourself sufficient time to rest and recover, and incorporate rest days or light activities into your routine to avoid overtraining and injuries.

9. Gradually Incorporate Plyometric Exercises:

- To enhance your power and explosiveness, incorporate plyometric exercises such as wall jump squats and wall burpees into your workout routine once you have established a strong foundation.
- When you first begin, begin with a lesser intensity and volume, and as your strength and endurance develop, progressively increase as you progress.

10. Seek Professional Guidance:

- To ensure that you are performing exercises with the correct form and technique, especially as you graduate to more complex exercises, you might think about working with a Pilates instructor or a fitness trainer.
- An expert can give you with individualized tweaks and variations that are tailored to your current fitness level and your desired outcomes.

Breathing Techniques

One of the most important aspects of the Pilates method is the concept of breathing. Joseph devoted a sizeable amount of the introduction to his book to breathing, which he referred to as the internal blood circulation-driven housecleaning that occurs within the body. Within this section, he provided an overview of his viewpoint regarding the relevance of increasing oxygen intake and circulation to all parts of the body. He regarded this as a process that was both rejuvenating and purifying.

When performing the various Pilates exercises, it is necessary to take slow, deep breaths and then release them at the appropriate time. This is the act of breathing. As was said before, the Pilates method requires an awareness of how the body works in order to be completed successfully. Breathing is the most important physical component that must be present in order to achieve that level of consciousness. If one breathes in the right way, they will be able to be in the present moment.

During the process of breathing, Joseph instructs us to visualize our lungs as bellows and to make use of them in a strong manner in order to propel air into and out of our bodies. For example, when you inhale, you are completely taking in air, and when you exhale, you are doing the same thing. He went so far as to assert that controlling one's breathing is the most important aspect of any and all activities, and that the first step is to become proficient in proper breathing techniques. In addition to this, he emphasized how essential it is to complete the Pilates exercises while taking a really deep breath.

A characteristic of the posterior lateral breathing technique utilized in Pilates is the practice of taking deep breaths into the back and sides of the rib cage. During the exhalation process, it is essential to pay attention to the contraction of the abdominal muscles and the pelvic floor muscles. When performing each exercise, Pilates makes an effort to coordinate this breathing pattern with the movement. During any of the exercises, the most crucial instruction is to ensure that you are breathing appropriately.

Due to the fact that it acts as a reminder to breathe correctly and to take deep breaths that are rich in oxygen, the principle of breathing is also extremely helpful in our day-to-day lives. It is general knowledge that breathing is the primary mechanism that maintains our bodily existence throughout our entire lives.

The concept of breathing also assists us in paying more attention to the emotional and physical happenings that are taking place in our immediate environment. In addition to reacting to it, we get a more profound awareness of it as a result of our experience. In the event that someone yells at you during an argument, for instance, the breathing principle permits you to take a deep breath and accurately assess the situation before reacting to them. As a consequence of this, you have more time to think about the situation and respond appropriately when such scenarios arise.

Flow

The Pilates exercises are executed in a manner that is fluid and steady. The goals of this principle are to achieve elegance, ease, fluidity, and smooth motions, all of which are essential for doing any kind of resistance training. During the process of transitioning between postures, the individual will experience an increase in their strength and endurance as a result of their fluid and continuous movement. During the course of the exercise, the energy must circulate through the body in a manner that is consistent and connected in order to facilitate the achievement of perfect integration. Pilates apparatus is a helpful tool that simulates attention and flow, similar to the Reformer, which is a traditional Pilates machine.

It is important to keep in mind that the actions become simpler when they are related with specific rhythms. The fundamental goal of this principle is to ensure that continuity is maintained throughout all actions, particularly when doing several repetitions. When you practice Pilates exercises with proper form, you improve your performance and lower your risk of injury.

Within the context of our day-to-day lives, the concept of flow urges us to accept things in their current state. The ability to accept life as it develops and moves through us on a daily basis creates opportunities for us. When people talk about living "in the flow" or "together with the flow," they are referring to the ability to navigate the many challenges and distractions that life presents without becoming easily distracted. In the same way, when we build rhythm and flow in our movements, our lives flow effortlessly as well. Through the practice of smooth transitions, we are able to successfully manage the many changes that occur in our lives.

Numerous changes and transitions occur in our lives on a daily basis as we continue to grow and develop. The activities that we do on a daily basis require a significant amount of energy, and if we are unable to effectively manage this energy and do all of our tasks without any trouble, we may experience difficulties.

Conclusion

"Wall Pilates Workouts for Women" has been a transformative, empowering, and rejuvenating experience. It's important to consider the major components that have influenced this book and how they support a holistic approach to fitness and well-being as we near the conclusion of this extensive guide. This epilogue seeks to distill the essence of the subjects discussed, restate the book's fulfillment of its promises, and highlight the main lesson that will stay with you long after the last page is turned.

"Wall Pilates Workouts for Women" set out to present a fresh and approachable type of exercise designed with women in mind from the very beginning. By combining the basic ideas of classical Pilates with the adaptability and support of a wall, wall Pilates creates an exercise setting that improves control, alignment, and stability. Exercises that are suitable for people of all fitness levels, from novices to experts, can be made possible by the wall's resistance and support capabilities.

The examination of Pilates' fundamental concepts—concentration, control, centering, precision, breath, and flow—was at the heart of this work. These ideas were covered in detail in each chapter, showing how they supported each and every Wall Pilates posture and movement. You have gained the ability to execute workouts with awareness and purpose, assuring optimal results and lowering the chance of harm, by internalizing these concepts.

Understanding anatomy and physiology in depth was necessary to fully comprehend the physical effects of Wall Pilates. This book offered thorough insights into the skeletal and muscular systems, highlighting the significance of muscular balance, spinal alignment, and core strength. Knowing which muscle groups are worked throughout various exercises gives you the ability to customize your workouts to meet your own needs and objectives.

"Wall Pilates Workouts for Women" is notable for its versatility, as it can be tailored to suit various phases of a woman's life. This book offers personalized workouts that cater to your unique physical and emotional demands, regardless of your age—young adult, working professional, new mother, or approaching retirement. The goal for young adults was to lay a solid foundation and avoid getting hurt again. The emphasis of the workouts was efficiency and stress alleviation for working professionals. While older women benefitted from workouts that enhance joint health and mobility, new mothers discovered regimens that support postpartum recovery.

Lifestyle decisions and diet are intrinsically linked to physical fitness. The significance of a well-rounded diet full of whole foods, staying hydrated, and getting enough sleep was emphasized in this book. In addition to your Pilates practice, nutritional assistance was given to make sure your body had the nourishment it needs to function and recuperate at its best. The book also covered lifestyle elements that are critical to achieving total well-being, like getting enough sleep, managing stress, and maintaining a happy outlook.

This book acknowledged that achieving fitness is frequently a difficult journey and provided helpful answers to typical roadblocks. You've been able to overcome obstacles like time restraints, low motivation, or physical limits thanks to the techniques that have been presented. In order to ensure long-term adherence and success, the focus was on developing a sustainable exercise regimen that blends effortlessly into your lifestyle.

Numerous testimonies and case studies demonstrated the life-changing impact of Wall Pilates across the chapters. Women from all walks of life reported experiencing better posture, stronger muscles, more flexibility, and sharper minds. These accounts demonstrated the ability of Wall Pilates to improve self-esteem and confidence in addition to changing the body.

"Wall Pilates Workouts for Women" promised to offer a complete, practical, and efficient exercise program designed with women in mind. This book has fulfilled its promise by providing a comprehensive strategy that incorporates lifestyle, diet, and exercise. With the help of the carefully designed exercises, which are supported by reliable scientific theories and enhanced by useful advice and inspirational stories, you may now reach your fitness objectives.

The most important lesson to remember when you end this book is the empowerment that results from regularity. Wall Pilates is a way of life, not merely an exercise program. You can get the advantages of better posture, strength, flexibility, and mental clarity with dedication and consistent practice. You are making a long-term investment in your health and wellbeing when you incorporate Wall Pilates into your regular practice.

Committing to write this book was a labor of love, motivated by my desire to share the transformative power of Pilates with women. You are on a path of self-improvement and self-discovery. Keep in mind that each stride, each movement, and each breath you take during your Wall Pilates practice will help you become a better, happier version of yourself. Accept the process, acknowledge your accomplishments, and never waver in your commitment to your fitness quest.

Although this book provides a thorough introduction to Wall Pilates, your adventure with it is far from ended. Keep trying out new workouts, push yourself with more difficult regimens, and maintain an open mind regarding your body's possibilities. Create a supportive community, share your experiences with others, and encourage people close to you to start their own fitness adventures.

Ultimately, "Wall Pilates Workouts for Women" has given you a solid foundation in Wall Pilates's tenets, techniques, and advantages. It has given you the information and resources you need to design a customized exercise program that meets your specific requirements and objectives. You may achieve the transformation you desire because it is driven by the ideas of empowerment, mindfulness, and constancy.

Take the main takeaway from this book with you as you proceed: fitness is a journey, not a destination. Accept the highs and lows, remain dedicated to your practice, and most importantly, have faith in your capacity to build and preserve a robust, balanced life. In your practice, the wall might serve as a prop, but your true strength lies within. Cheers to your ongoing success and health as you embark on this lifelong Wall Pilates journey.

Printed in Great Britain
by Amazon